HERBAL REMEDIES FOR DIABETES CONTROL

Nourishing A Comprehensive Guide to Diabetes Through **Nature's Pharmacy**

Tara Wason

CONTENTS

Introduction...**5**

UNDERSTANDING DIABETES: TYPES, CAUSES, AND SYMPTOMS...........................9

VARIETIES OF DIABETES...9

ROOT CAUSES OF DIABETES..11

INDICATORS OF DIABETES..13

HERBAL APPROACH TO DIABETES: UNVEILING TRADITION AND SCIENCE..............**16**

HERITAGE OF HERBAL USE..17

SCIENTIFIC INSIGHTS INTO HERBAL REMEDIES....................................19

INTEGRATION OF HERBAL FORMULAS IN MODERN CONTEXT.......................21

CHALLENGES AND FUTURE PROSPECTS...23

KEY HERBS FOR DIABETES CONTROL...**25**

FUTURE HORIZONS AND RESEARCH AVENUES.......................................32

HERBAL RECIPES AND FORMULAS..**35**

HERBAL TEAS...35

TINCTURES AND EXTRACTS..39

COOKING WITH DIABETES-FRIENDLY HERBS..42

CULINARY CONSIDERATIONS AND WELLNESS SYNERGIES..........................46

FUTURE HORIZONS..47

EMBRACING A HEALTHFUL LIFESTYLE...**49**

THE ESSENTIAL ROLE OF EXERCISE IN DIABETES MANAGEMENT....................49

TAILORING EXERCISE TO INDIVIDUAL NEEDS......................................52

ADVICE ON CULTIVATING HEALTHY EATING HABITS..............................53

INTEGRATING HERBS WITH STANDARD TREATMENTS..............................**59**

NAVIGATING POSSIBLE INTERACTIONS AND SAFETY MEASURES....................59

COLLABORATIVE APPROACHES FOR IMPROVED THERAPEUTIC OUTCOMES...........63

EXPLORING HERB-DRUG COMBINATIONS FOR SPECIFIC HEALTH CONDITIONS.........**68**

ADDRESSING CHALLENGES AND MAXIMIZING BENEFITS.............................71

Future Frontiers: Advances in Integrative Healthcare......74

A Thorough Guide to Ethical Herbal Utilisation...... 78

Grasping Responsible Herbal Utilization...... 78

The Imperative of Seeking Professional Guidance...... 82

Adhering to Safety Guidelines: A Shared Responsibility......85

Promoting Education and Empowerment...... 87

Regulatory Compliance and Quality Assurance......88

Crafting Your Personalized Herbal Diabetes Toolkit......91

Developing Your Unique Herbal Plan...... 91

Reliable Sources for Obtaining Premium-Quality Herbs......95

FAQs on Herbal Remedies for Diabetes...... 102

Grasping Diabetes and the Role of Herbal Solutions...... 102

Varieties, Causes, and Symptoms of Diabetes...... 104

Efficacy and Safety of Herbal Remedies...... 106

Integrating Herbal Remedies into Daily Life......108

Addressing Challenges and Taking Precautions...... 110

Herbal Remedies: Beyond Blood Sugar Control...... 112

Future Avenues and Research...... 113

Conclusion...... 116

Embracing Holistic Diabetes Management...... 122

Introduction

In providing a succinct exploration of diabetes, it becomes imperative to delineate the multifaceted nature of this metabolic disorder. Diabetes, a prevalent health condition, manifests in distinct types, each characterized by irregularities in insulin production or utilization. While Type 1 diabetes stems from the body's inability to produce insulin, Type 2 diabetes arises from inadequate insulin utilization, often associated with lifestyle factors. This chronic ailment is marked by elevated blood glucose levels, leading to a range of complications affecting vital organs and systems.

Within the realm of diabetes management, a noteworthy avenue deserving attention is the realm of natural remedies. Amid the myriad approaches available, the significance of embracing nature's pharmacy emerges prominently. Natural remedies, rooted in traditional practices and substantiated by scientific inquiry, offer a holistic perspective on diabetes control. Unlike conventional pharmaceutical interventions, these remedies harness the inherent therapeutic properties of various herbs and plants, presenting an alternative that not only complements but enhances the overall wellness journey.

The significance of turning to natural remedies lies not only in their historical efficacy but also in their potential to address the root causes of diabetes. Embracing herbal solutions aligns with the body's intrinsic processes, promoting balance and mitigating the adverse effects of the condition. As we embark on this exploration of herbal remedies for diabetes control, the intention is to illuminate a path that not only manages symptoms but fosters a symbiotic relationship between individuals and the botanical resources bestowed by nature. Through this, we embark on a journey that converges traditional wisdom with contemporary scientific validation, offering a nuanced perspective on fostering health and well-being amidst the complexities of diabetes.

Understanding Diabetes: Types, Causes, and Symptoms

Diabetes, a widespread metabolic disorder characterized by elevated blood glucose levels, demands a comprehensive grasp of its distinct types, underlying causes, and presenting symptoms for effective management and prevention.

Varieties of Diabetes

Type 1 Diabetes

Diagnosed typically in childhood or adolescence, Type 1 diabetes stems from an autoimmune assault on pancreatic beta cells, resulting in insufficient insulin production.

Genetic predispositions and environmental triggers contribute to the intricate origins of this type.

Type 2 Diabetes

In contrast, Type 2 diabetes, more prevalent and typically occurring later in life, associates with insulin resistance and impaired insulin secretion. Lifestyle factors, including sedentary habits and dietary choices, significantly impact the onset and progression of Type 2 diabetes.

Gestational Diabetes

A transient condition during pregnancy, gestational diabetes heightens the risk of

Type 2 diabetes later in life. Inadequate insulin production in response to increased pregnancy-related demands underscores the importance of effective management.

Root Causes of Diabetes

1. Genetic Influences

Genetic factors play a substantial role in diabetes susceptibility, with certain gene variants contributing to a predisposition for the condition. Family history often indicates the hereditary aspect of diabetes.

2. Environmental Triggers

Sedentary lifestyles and unhealthy dietary patterns are prominent environmental factors influencing diabetes. The prevalence of processed foods rich in refined sugars and unhealthy fats amplifies the risk of insulin resistance and Type 2 diabetes.

3. Autoimmune Responses

In Type 1 diabetes, an autoimmune response prompts the immune system to mistakenly target and destroy pancreatic beta cells. Investigations into the triggers for this response point to a combination of genetic and environmental factors.

Indicators of Diabetes

1. Excessive Urination and Thirst

Characteristic symptoms of diabetes include polyuria (excessive urination) and polydipsia (excessive thirst). Elevated blood glucose levels lead to increased urine production, causing dehydration and heightened thirst.

2. Unintended Weight Loss

Despite increased hunger, unintended weight loss is a common symptom. The body, unable to utilize glucose efficiently, resorts to breaking down fats and proteins for energy, resulting in weight loss.

3. Fatigue and Weakness

Persistently elevated blood glucose levels induce fatigue and weakness. The compromised ability to utilize glucose affects energy production, leading to a constant sense of tiredness.

4. Vision Disturbances

Diabetes impacts the eyes, causing blurred vision. Fluctuating blood glucose levels contribute to changes in the eye's lens shape, affecting visual clarity.

5. Delayed Wound Healing

Impaired blood circulation and compromised immune function in diabetes slow down the healing process. Wounds and infections take longer to heal, increasing the risk of complications.

Concluding Insights

A holistic understanding of diabetes involves recognizing its diverse types, comprehending the intricate interplay of genetic and environmental factors in its causation, and remaining vigilant to the array of symptoms that may manifest. This knowledge forms the basis for effective prevention, management, and ongoing research efforts aimed at unravelling the complexities of this prevalent metabolic disorder.

Herbal Approach to Diabetes: Unveiling Tradition and Science

The historical application of herbs in diabetes care has deep roots, steeped in the annals of traditional medicine, presenting a tapestry of wisdom. Simultaneously, contemporary scientific inquiry has illuminated the intricate mechanisms underlying the effectiveness of herbal remedies, providing a robust basis for incorporating nature's pharmacopeia into the management of diabetes.

Heritage of Herbal Use

- Ancient Healing Traditions

Across diverse cultures, the utilization of herbs for addressing health concerns, including diabetes, has been a longstanding practice. Ancient healing systems, from Ayurveda to Traditional Chinese Medicine, embraced various botanical remedies to restore equilibrium within the body.

- Traditional Herbal Blends

Drawing on generations of experiential knowledge, herbalists and healers crafted sophisticated formulas, incorporating revered botanicals like bitter melon, fenugreek seeds, and cinnamon. These blends aimed to alleviate diabetes symptoms and revitalize overall well-being.

- Cultural Embedment

The historical use of herbs was deeply embedded in cultural practices, becoming integral to rituals and traditions. The transmission of herbal knowledge across generations underscored the pivotal role of these natural remedies in promoting well-being.

Scientific Insights into Herbal Remedies

- Potency of Phytochemicals

Modern scientific scrutiny has unveiled the potent bioactive compounds within herbs, termed phytochemicals, which confer therapeutic benefits. Compounds such as flavonoids and polyphenols exhibit anti-diabetic properties, influencing glucose metabolism and insulin sensitivity.

- Mechanisms of Operation

Herbal remedies operate through diverse mechanisms, impacting insulin production, release, and cellular responses to glucose. The interplay of botanical compounds with cellular signalling pathways provides a nuanced understanding of how herbs contribute to managing diabetes.

- Antioxidant Defense

Many herbs possess robust antioxidant properties, alleviating oxidative stress—a hallmark of diabetes complications. By neutralizing free radicals, herbs contribute to cellular protection, mitigating vascular and neurological issues associated with diabetes.

Integration of Herbal Formulas in Modern Context

Complementing Conventional Treatments

In contemporary diabetes care, there's a growing acknowledgment of the synergy between herbal remedies and conventional treatments. Rather than being viewed as alternatives, herbs are seen as complementary agents, enhancing the overall effectiveness of diabetes management.

Evidence-Based Validation

Increasingly, scientific studies and clinical trials validate the efficacy of specific herbs in controlling diabetes. From influencing blood glucose levels to improving lipid profiles, the expanding evidence base supports the integration of herbal interventions into mainstream healthcare.

Personalized Approaches

The herbal approach to diabetes underscores personalized interventions, recognizing individual responses to botanical compounds. Tailoring herbal formulas to an individual's constitution and diabetes profile emphasizes the holistic nature of this approach.

Challenges and Future Prospects
Standardization and Quality Control

Ensuring standardized formulations and rigorous quality control presents a challenge for the herbal approach. Consistency in herbal products is crucial for both safety and efficacy.

Collaborative Synergy

The collaboration between traditional herbal wisdom and modern scientific methodologies offers promising prospects for future research. Bridging the gap between ancestral knowledge and contemporary scientific rigor holds the key to unlocking the full potential of herbal interventions in diabetes care.

Concluding Insights

Exploring the herbal approach to diabetes navigates a continuum intertwining historical botanical remedies with modern scientific scrutiny. The synergy between tradition and science invites exploration, understanding, and harnessing the healing potential nature provides in diabetes management. Amidst this intricate landscape, the herbal approach stands as a testament to the enduring relevance of ancient wisdom in shaping the future landscape of healthcare.

Key Herbs for Diabetes Control

The domain of herbal remedies for diabetes control encompasses a diverse array of botanical allies that have played pivotal roles in both traditional and modern approaches. This exploration delves into the unique attributes of **Aloe vera, Bitter melon, Fenugreek, Cinnamon, Gymnema Sylvestre, and Turmeric**, shedding light on their individual contributions to the management of diabetes.

1. Aloe vera

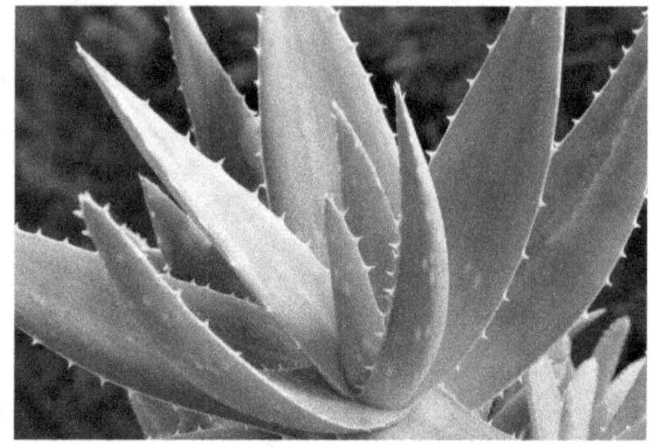

Aloe vera, esteemed for its versatile healing properties, extends its benefits to diabetes care. Abundant in bioactive compounds, it aids in lowering blood glucose levels and enhancing insulin sensitivity. The gel extracted from Aloe vera leaves holds potential in alleviating diabetic complications and fostering overall well-being.

2. Bitter Melon

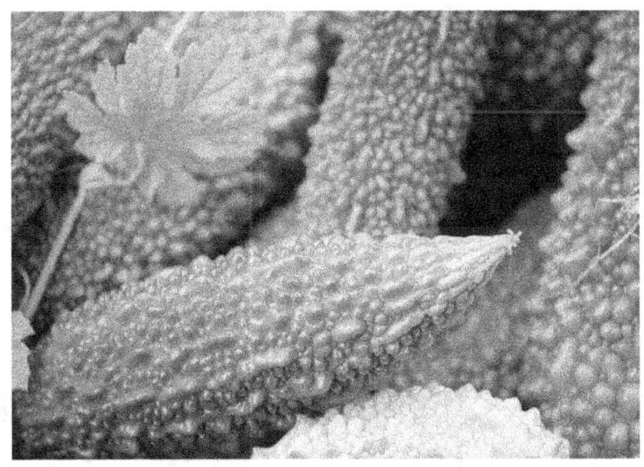

Bitter melon, a staple in various traditional medicines, emerges as a potent botanical ally in diabetes control. Its active compounds, including charantin and polypeptide-p, mimic insulin effects, facilitating glucose uptake. Additionally, bitter melon showcases antioxidant properties, contributing to the prevention of complications associated with diabetes.

3. Fenugreek

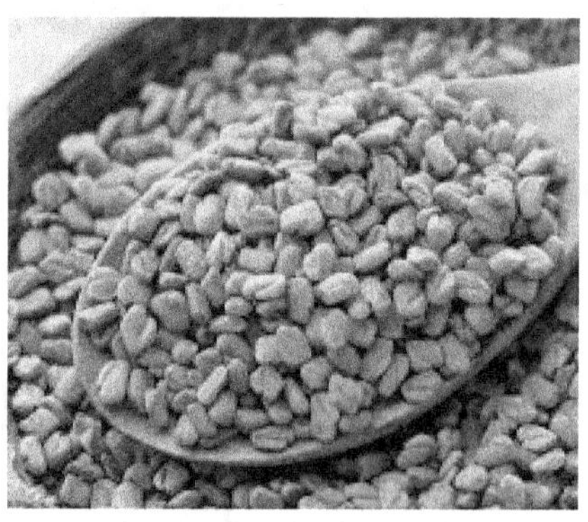

Fenugreek seeds, renowned for both culinary and medicinal uses, stand out as potent regulators of glycemia. Laden with soluble fibre and hypoglycaemic compounds, fenugreek aids in controlling blood sugar levels, improving insulin sensitivity, and enhancing lipid profiles. Its adaptability in both culinary applications and herbal formulations underscores its significance in diabetes management.

4. Cinnamon

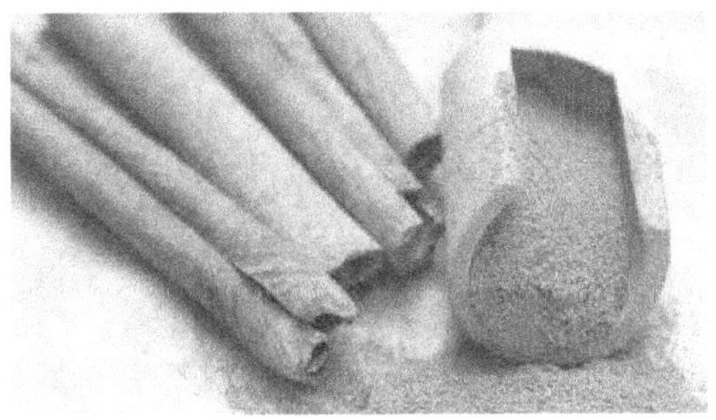

Cinnamon, beyond its culinary allure, emerges as a spice with therapeutic potential in diabetes care. Active components, particularly cinnamaldehyde, boost insulin sensitivity, facilitate glucose uptake, and counteract oxidative stress. Whether integrated into dietary practices or used as a supplement, cinnamon holds promise in supporting the regulation of blood sugar.

5. Gymnema Sylvestre

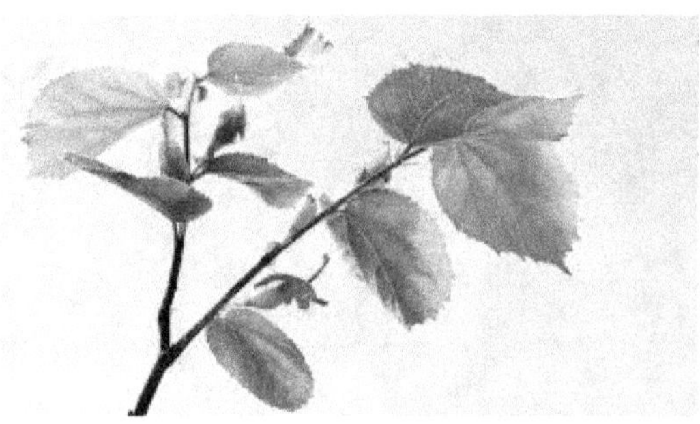

Gymnema Sylvestre, aptly dubbed the "sugar destroyer," boasts a longstanding reputation in Ayurvedic medicine for its anti-diabetic properties. Gymnemic acids within it block sugar absorption in the intestines and stimulate the regeneration of pancreatic beta cells, contributing to enhanced insulin production. The role of Gymnema Sylvestre in curbing sugar cravings further accentuates its potential in diabetes control.

6. Turmeric

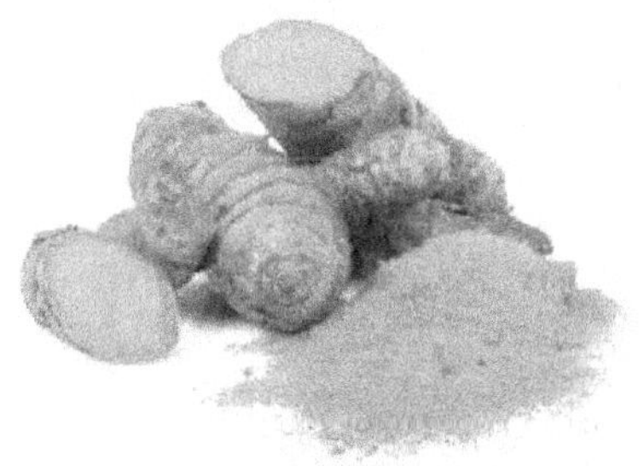

Turmeric, the revered golden spice renowned for its anti-inflammatory and antioxidant properties, proves to be a versatile contributor to diabetes management. Its active compound, curcumin, displays anti-diabetic effects by improving insulin sensitivity, reducing inflammation, and safeguarding against diabetic complications. Whether incorporated into culinary practices or consumed as a supplement, turmeric enriches the holistic approach to diabetes care.

Future Horizons and Research Avenues

While these key herbs exhibit promise in diabetes control, ongoing research endeavours persist in unveiling their complete potential. Exploring the synergies between traditional wisdom and contemporary scientific methodologies remains essential for unlocking new dimensions in herbal interventions for diabetes care.

Concluding Insights

In uncovering the distinctive contributions of Aloe vera, Bitter melon, Fenugreek, Cinnamon, Gymnema Sylvestre, and Turmeric, I reveal a herbal mosaic that enriches the tapestry of diabetes management. From ancient roots to contemporary applications, these key herbs embody the symbiotic relationship between nature's bounty and the pursuit of holistic well-being within the domain of diabetes care.

Herbal Recipes and Formulas

In the pursuit of holistic health, herbal recipes and formulas present a delightful avenue, offering not only therapeutic advantages but also a rich culinary experience. This exploration delves into the realms of herbal teas, the crafting of tinctures and extracts, and the seamless integration of diabetes-friendly herbs into the culinary realm.

Herbal Teas

Creating a Calming Aloe Vera Infusion

Aloe vera, known for its healing properties, can be incorporated into a soothing herbal infusion. By steeping either fresh aloe vera gel or dried leaves in hot water, a gentle and hydrating tea is produced, offering a refreshing option with potential benefits for digestion and blood sugar balance.

Bitter Melon Elixir

Bitter melon, a revered ingredient in traditional medicine, reveals its potential in a therapeutic tea. Slices of bitter melon fruit, steeped in hot water, create an elixir rich in charantin and polypeptide-p, providing not just a distinctive taste but also potential benefits for regulating blood sugar.

Fenugreek Infusion

Versatile fenugreek seeds transform into a fragrant herbal infusion. By simmering these seeds in hot water, a tea rich in soluble fibre and hypoglycaemic compounds emerges, offering a delightful way to support glycaemic control.

Cinnamon Spice Tea

Cinnamon, beyond its culinary appeal, imparts its aromatic delight to a therapeutic tea. Boiling cinnamon sticks or ground cinnamon in water produces a warming infusion, not only adding a pleasant flavour but also potentially aiding insulin sensitivity and glucose regulation.

Gymnema sylvestre Elixir

Gymnema sylvestre, known as the "sugar destroyer," takes centre stage in an herbal elixir. By steeping gymnema leaves in hot water, a tea is created that may contribute to reducing sugar cravings, making it a flavourful ally in diabetes management.

Turmeric Golden Tea

Golden turmeric introduces its anti-inflammatory and antioxidant properties into a versatile tea. Simmering turmeric, ginger, and black pepper in water creates a vibrant concoction, offering not only a comforting beverage but also potential anti-diabetic benefits.

Aloe Vera Tincture

Aloe vera's healing potential is intensified in a concentrated tincture. By soaking aloe vera leaves in alcohol or glycerin, a potent extract is created, capturing the therapeutic essence for potential use in skincare or internal consumption.

Bitter Melon Extract

The unique bitterness of bitter melon is concentrated in an herbal extract. By soaking bitter melon slices in alcohol or vinegar, an extract rich in bioactive compounds emerges, offering a versatile elixir with potential benefits for blood sugar regulation.

Fenugreek Tincture

The nutritional richness of fenugreek finds concentration in a tincture. By immersing fenugreek seeds in alcohol, a potent extract is obtained, preserving the herb's medicinal properties for potential use in supporting glycaemic control.

Cinnamon Essence Extract

The aromatic essence of cinnamon is captured in a concentrated extract. By infusing cinnamon in alcohol or glycerin, a versatile extract is crafted, offering a potent addition to various recipes with potential anti-diabetic properties.

Gymnema Sylvestre Solution

Gymnema Sylvestre's "sugar destroyer" qualities are harnessed in a liquid solution. By steeping gymnema leaves in alcohol or glycerin, a concentrated extract is produced, presenting a convenient way to incorporate this herb's potential benefits into daily routines.

Turmeric Elixir

The golden brilliance of turmeric is preserved in a concentrated elixir. By infusing turmeric in alcohol or glycerin, a versatile extract is formed, offering a convenient means to introduce anti-inflammatory and anti-diabetic properties into various culinary creations.

Cooking with Diabetes-Friendly Herbs

Aloe Vera Culinary Marvels: From Salads to Smoothies

Aloe vera's culinary versatility shines in various dishes. Incorporating fresh aloe vera gel into salads or blending it into smoothies not only adds a refreshing touch but also introduces potential health benefits, making it an innovative approach to culinary creations.

Bitter Melon Gastronomic Adventure: Stir-Fries and Soups

Bitter melon, traditionally admired in culinary realms, finds a place in stir-fries and soups. Sautéed or simmered, bitter melon adds a unique flavour profile while potentially contributing to glycaemic control, presenting a delightful culinary adventure.

Fenugreek Culinary Harmony: From Curries to Breads

Fenugreek seeds, a staple in culinary traditions, lend their aromatic harmony to curries and bread. Whether toasted in curries or incorporated into bread recipes, fenugreek introduces a distinctive taste while offering potential benefits for glycemic regulation.

Cinnamon Infused Delights: Baked Treasures and Morning Oats

Cinnamon's aromatic charm permeates baked treats and morning oats. From cinnamon-infused cookies to oatmeal sprinkled with this spice, the culinary landscape becomes not only delightful but also potentially supportive of blood sugar management.

Gymnema Sylvestre Culinary Fusion: Soups and Stews

Gymnema Sylvestre seamlessly blends into soups and stews. Simmered alongside other herbs and spices, it imparts its unique essence while potentially contributing to sugar cravings management, adding a nuanced layer to culinary creations.

Turmeric Culinary Elevation: Golden Soups and Curries

Turmeric's golden hue elevates soups and curries. Whether in a hearty soup or a spiced curry, turmeric not only enhances the visual appeal but also introduces anti-inflammatory and potential anti-diabetic qualities into culinary masterpieces.

Culinary Considerations and Wellness Synergies

Embarking on this culinary journey, infusing herbal teas, crafting tinctures and extracts, and seamlessly incorporating diabetes-friendly herbs into cooking, reveals a symphony of flavours. Recognizing the unique attributes of each herb and understanding the potential synergies in combining them forms the basis for a holistic approach to wellness through culinary arts.

Future Horizons

While these herbal recipes and formulas showcase promise in both flavour and potential health benefits, ongoing exploration and scientific inquiry continue to unveil new dimensions. The intersection between traditional culinary wisdom and modern nutritional science paves the way for innovative culinary creations that contribute not only to the palate but also to holistic well-being.

Concluding Insights

Navigating the realms of herbal teas, crafting tinctures and extracts, and seamlessly incorporating diabetes-friendly herbs into cooking, unfolds a rich culinary tapestry. From traditional roots to modern kitchens, these practices embody the harmonious relationship between nature's bounty and the pursuit of holistic well-being within the context of diabetes care.

Embracing a Healthful Lifestyle

Effective diabetes management extends beyond medications, encompassing critical aspects of lifestyle and dietary choices. This exploration delves into the pivotal role of exercise in diabetes care and provides advice on adopting healthful eating habits, offering a holistic guide for individuals navigating the complex landscape of diabetes.

The Essential Role of Exercise in Diabetes Management

Exercise is a fundamental element in managing diabetes, serving as a potent supporter in controlling blood sugar levels.

Regular physical activity improves insulin sensitivity, facilitating efficient glucose utilization by cells, not only regulating blood sugar but also contributing to overall metabolic health.

i.   Aerobic Exercise

Incorporating aerobic exercises like brisk walking, jogging, or cycling is a crucial strategy. These activities elevate heart rate, promoting cardiovascular health, enhancing blood circulation, and aiding glucose transport to cells. The cumulative benefits extend beyond diabetes management to encompass broader well-being.

ii.   Resistance Training

Engaging in resistance training, including activities like weightlifting, contributes to building muscle mass and enhancing insulin sensitivity. As muscles play a key role in glucose metabolism, their improved function aids in maintaining stable blood sugar levels, addressing metabolic intricacies linked with diabetes.

iii.   Flexibility and Balance Exercises

Holistic well-being is fostered through flexibility and balance exercises. Activities like yoga or tai chi not only enhance physical flexibility but also promote balance, reducing the risk of falls—a crucial consideration for individuals with diabetes facing complications related to neuropathy.

Tailoring Exercise to Individual Needs

Acknowledging that exercise is not one-size-fits-all, customizing physical activity to individual preferences and health conditions is vital. Consultation with healthcare professionals and fitness experts helps design personalized exercise regimens aligned with both specific diabetes management requirements and individual lifestyles.

Advice on Cultivating Healthy Eating Habits

- Embracing a Balanced Diet

Healthy eating forms the foundation of diabetes management. A balanced diet, incorporating a variety of nutrient-dense foods, regulates blood sugar levels and supports overall health. Prioritizing a mix of carbohydrates, proteins, fats, vitamins, and minerals ensures sustained energy levels and nutritional adequacy.

- Carbohydrate Management

Carbohydrates play a crucial role in blood sugar regulation, requiring a nuanced approach to consumption. Prioritizing complex carbohydrates with a low glycaemic index, such as whole grains, legumes, and vegetables, stabilizes blood sugar levels. Portion control and mindful eating optimize carbohydrate management.

- Protein-Rich Foods

Incorporating lean protein sources, such as poultry, fish, tofu, and legumes, supports muscle health and provides a lasting feeling of fullness. This aids in weight management and contributes to blood sugar control, as proteins have a minimal impact on glycaemic levels.

- Healthy Fats Lipid

Choosing healthy fats, such as those found in avocados, nuts, and olive oil, promotes cardiovascular health and complements diabetes management. Balancing fat intake and avoiding excessive saturated and trans fats align with dietary guidelines optimizing lipid profiles.

- Mindful Eating Practices

Cultivating mindfulness in eating involves savouring each bite, recognizing hunger and fullness cues, and avoiding distractions during meals. This mindful approach fosters a healthier relationship with food, promoting better digestion and aiding in weight management—key components of diabetes care.

- Hydration

Adequate hydration, often overlooked, holds significant importance in diabetes management. Water consumption supports kidney function, regulates blood sugar levels, and aids overall metabolic processes. Choosing water over sugary beverages aligns with dietary guidelines for both diabetes and general health.

Concluding insights

In navigating the intricate landscape of diabetes care, embracing a holistic lifestyle that intertwines regular exercise and healthful eating habits emerges as a powerful strategy. From the physiological benefits of physical activity to the nuanced considerations in dietary choices, this comprehensive guide offers insights and guidance for individuals seeking to optimize their well-being while living with diabetes. The synergy between lifestyle choices, medical interventions, and ongoing support creates a robust foundation for a fulfilling and healthy life with diabetes.

Integrating Herbs with Standard Treatments

The convergence of conventional medicinal approaches and traditional herbal remedies provides a holistic avenue for well-being. This examination delves into the precautions and potential interactions associated with combining herbs and standard treatments, while also revealing collaborative methods to enhance therapeutic results.

Navigating Possible Interactions and Safety Measures

- Grasping Herb-Drug Dynamics

Blending herbs with conventional medications demands a nuanced comprehension of potential interactions. Certain herbs can influence drug metabolism, affecting how pharmaceuticals are absorbed, distributed, metabolized, and excreted. Being aware of these interactions is critical to preventing adverse effects and optimizing treatment results.

- Acknowledging Individual Variability

Responses to combinations of herbs and drugs differ among individuals due to factors like genetics, overall health, and existing medical conditions. Customizing treatment plans to individual needs requires a thorough understanding of these variables, ensuring a tailored approach that minimizes risks and maximizes therapeutic advantages.

- Monitoring for Adverse Effects and Adjusting Treatments

Vigilant monitoring for side effects is essential when merging herbs with conventional treatments. Regular assessments, such as blood tests and clinical evaluations, aid in promptly identifying any adverse reactions. Collaborative adjustments to treatment plans between healthcare providers and individuals ensure a balanced and secure therapeutic strategy.

- Special Considerations for Vulnerable Populations

Certain populations, such as pregnant women, the elderly, and individuals with pre-existing health conditions, may require extra precautions. Healthcare professionals should exercise heightened vigilance and factor in potential herb-drug interactions within the context of individual health conditions.

Establishing Transparent Communication with Healthcare Providers

Effective integration hinges on transparent communication between individuals and healthcare providers. Open discussions regarding herb usage, conventional medications, and health objectives foster a collaborative atmosphere where treatment plans can be tailored to individual needs while minimizing potential risks.

Comprehensive Health Assessments for Informed Decision-Making

Informed decision-making relies on comprehensive health assessments that consider medical history, lifestyle factors, and existing treatment regimens. Merging herbal remedies into conventional treatments requires a holistic understanding of an individual's health profile, enabling healthcare providers to make well-informed recommendations.

Gradual Integration for Controlled Adaptation

A gradual approach to integrating herbs with conventional treatments often proves beneficial. Introducing herbal remedies slowly allows for controlled adaptation, enabling healthcare providers to monitor individual responses and make adjustments as necessary. This methodical integration minimizes the risk of abrupt changes and enhances the potential for therapeutic synergy.

Personalized Treatment Plans for Optimal Outcomes

Customizing treatment plans to individual needs is paramount for optimal results. Personalization involves considering an individual's health goals, preferences, and responsiveness to specific herbs. This collaborative and personalized approach ensures that the combined treatment strategy aligns with the individual's overall well-being.

Informed Consent and Individual Empowerment

Informed consent is a critical aspect of collaborative approaches. Individuals should be provided with comprehensive information regarding potential herb-drug interactions, expected outcomes, and any associated risks. This transparency enables individuals to actively participate in decisions concerning their treatment journey.

Exploring Herb-Drug Combinations for Specific Health Conditions

Managing Diabetes

The integration of herbs like bitter melon, fenugreek, and cinnamon with antidiabetic medications requires careful consideration. Bitter melon, known for potential hypoglycaemic effects, may enhance the actions of antidiabetic drugs. Fenugreek, with its impact on glucose metabolism, requires cautious integration. Cinnamon, recognized for potential benefits in insulin sensitivity, requires vigilant monitoring when combined with antidiabetic medications.

Cardiovascular Health

In the realm of cardiovascular health, herbs like hawthorn, garlic, and turmeric may exhibit interactions with heart medications. Hawthorn, known for potential cardiovascular benefits, may impact blood pressure medications. Garlic, recognized for potential anticoagulant effects, warrants careful consideration when combined with blood-thinning medications. Turmeric, celebrated for anti-inflammatory properties, may interact with certain heart medications, necessitating collaborative management.

Mental Health

In mental health, herbs like St. John's Wort and chamomile may interact with psychotropic medications. St. John's Wort, known for potential antidepressant effects, may impact the efficacy of certain antidepressant medications. Chamomile, celebrated for its calming properties, may interact with medications used for anxiety or sleep disorders. A collaborative approach is crucial in ensuring mental health treatments are optimized while minimizing potential risks.

Addressing Challenges and Maximizing Benefits

Tackling Information Discrepancies

Challenges in combining herbs with conventional treatments often arise from disparities in information. Not all individuals may disclose their herbal supplement use, and healthcare providers may not consistently inquire about herbal remedies. Bridging these information gaps requires proactive communication and comprehensive health assessments.

Education and Training for Healthcare Providers

Enhancing the education and training of healthcare providers on herbal remedies is pivotal. Integrative medicine courses and ongoing professional development can equip healthcare professionals with the knowledge needed to navigate herb-drug interactions and collaborate effectively with individuals seeking combined therapies.

Research and Evidence-Based Practices

Promoting research into herb-drug interactions and evidence-based practices is essential for advancing safe integration. Robust studies exploring the pharmacokinetics and pharmacodynamics of herb-drug combinations contribute to the development of guidelines and protocols, fostering a scientific foundation for collaborative approaches.

Patient Support Groups and Community Engagement

Creating patient support groups and fostering community engagement enhances shared knowledge and experiences. Peer support platforms provide individuals with spaces to share insights, challenges, and successes related to combining herbs with conventional treatments. This collaborative community approach contributes to a collective understanding of best practices.

Future Frontiers: Advances in Integrative Healthcare

Advances in Pharmacogenomics

Pharmacogenomics, exploring the genetic factors influencing individual responses to medications and herbs, holds promise for advancing integrative healthcare. Tailoring treatment plans based on genetic markers contributes to precision medicine, optimizing therapeutic outcomes and minimizing risks associated with herb-drug interactions.

Interdisciplinary Collaborations for Holistic Care

Interdisciplinary collaborations among healthcare providers, including herbalists, naturopaths, and conventional medical professionals, pave the way for holistic patient care. Shared knowledge, collaborative decision-making, and integrated treatment plans contribute to a comprehensive approach that addresses individual health from various perspectives.

Concluding insights

In the intricate interplay between herbs and conventional treatments, a synergistic approach emerges as a pathway to holistic well-being. Navigating potential interactions and precautions demands informed decision-making and open communication. Collaborative approaches, anchored in comprehensive assessments and personalized plans, optimize therapeutic outcomes. As we venture into the future, advancements in research and interdisciplinary collaborations hold the key to unlocking the full potential of integrative healthcare, fostering a landscape where the union of tradition and modernity becomes a powerful force for individual well-being.

A Thorough Guide to Ethical Herbal Utilisation

Embarking on the herbal remedies journey demands a nuanced grasp of safety precautions. In this comprehensive exploration, we delve into essential guidance for responsible herbal use, underlining the crucial necessity of consulting healthcare professionals throughout this endeavour.

Grasping Responsible Herbal Utilization

1. Herb Selection and Procurement: Commencing with Care

Commencing the journey involves meticulous herb selection and procurement. Individuals are advised to obtain herbs from trustworthy sources, ensuring both quality and adherence to ethical standards. Conducting thorough research into herb origins contributes to responsible usage, establishing a secure and effective foundation for the herbal approach.

2. Dosage Management: Achieving Equilibrium

Responsible herbal use centres around precise dosage considerations. Grasping the recommended dosages for specific herbs is crucial. Individuals are urged to diligently follow guidelines, avoiding the assumption that higher doses yield superior results.

Achieving a balance between therapeutic effects and potential risks is essential for maintaining safety.

3. Individual Response: Recognizing Uniqueness

Given that individual responses to herbs vary due to factors such as genetics and overall health, responsible herbal use necessitates acknowledgment of this variability. Tailoring herbal regimens to individual needs and closely monitoring responses contributes to a personalized approach that maximizes benefits while minimizing potential risks.

4. Duration of Use: Moderation as a Guiding Principle

Responsible herbal use involves moderation in the duration of use. Prolonged and excessive consumption of certain herbs may lead to unforeseen consequences. Establishing clear timelines for herbal regimens, coupled with periodic breaks, allows individuals to assess their responses and make informed decisions regarding continued use.

5. Herb Combinations: Navigating Complex Interactions

The combination of herbs demands careful consideration. Responsible use entails thorough research into potential herb-herb interactions, emphasizing transparency with healthcare providers to navigate complexities and ensure a harmonious integration.

The Imperative of Seeking Professional Guidance

1. Collaborative Decision-Making: A Partnership for Wellness

The cornerstone of responsible herbal use is collaborative decision-making with healthcare professionals. Establishing open lines of communication, sharing herbal regimens, and seeking guidance ensures that herbal approaches align with overall health goals and existing medical conditions.

2. Healthcare Provider Expertise: Drawing on Professional Knowledge

Harnessing the expertise of healthcare providers is instrumental in responsible herbal use. Professionals possess comprehensive knowledge of individual health profiles, enabling them to offer tailored advice on herb selection, dosage, and potential interactions with conventional medications.

3. Monitoring and Adjustments: A Dynamic Approach

Regular monitoring by healthcare professionals is a vital component of responsible herbal use. Ongoing assessments allow for adjustments to herbal regimens based on individual responses, ensuring a responsive and personalized healthcare strategy.

4. Pre-existing Conditions: Special Considerations

Individuals with pre-existing health conditions require special considerations in herbal use. Transparent communication with healthcare providers about existing medical conditions and ongoing treatments ensures that herbal approaches align with overall health management.

Adhering to Safety Guidelines: A Shared Responsibility

1. Adverse Reactions: Prompt Recognition and Response

Responsible herbal use entails prompt recognition and response to adverse reactions. Individuals are encouraged to be vigilant about changes in their well-being and report any unexpected symptoms to healthcare professionals.

2. Pregnancy and Lactation: Heightened Caution

Special precautions are essential for individuals who are pregnant or lactating. Responsible herbal use in these circumstances involves heightened caution, with healthcare providers guiding the selection of herbs that pose minimal risks.

3. Pediatric Considerations: Tailoring Approaches for Children

The use of herbs in pediatric populations necessitates tailored approaches. Responsible herbal use for children involves consulting healthcare providers for guidance on suitable herbs, dosages, and potential interactions.

Promoting Education and Empowerment
1. Individual Empowerment: Informed Decision-Making

Empowering individuals with knowledge is fundamental to responsible herbal use. Informed decision-making involves educating individuals about the properties, potential benefits, and risks associated with specific herbs.

2. Public Awareness: Fostering Informed Communities

Responsible herbal use extends to fostering public awareness. Initiatives that educate communities about the safe and informed use of herbs contribute to a collective understanding.

Regulatory Compliance and Quality Assurance

1. Regulatory Standards: Adhering to Guidelines

Responsible herbal use aligns with regulatory standards and guidelines. Individuals are encouraged to choose herbal products that comply with established regulations, ensuring quality, safety, and efficacy.

2. Quality Control: Ensuring Purity and Potency

Quality control measures are paramount in responsible herbal use. Individuals should prioritize herbs that undergo rigorous testing for purity and potency.

Concluding insight

In conclusion, responsible herbal use is anchored in a holistic approach that prioritizes individual well-being, collaborative decision-making with healthcare professionals, adherence to safety guidelines, and ongoing education. Navigating the world of herbal remedies with prudence and care allows individuals to harness the potential benefits of herbs while safeguarding against potential risks. Responsible herbal use emerges as a shared responsibility, promoting a harmonious integration of herbs into holistic healthcare strategies.

Crafting Your Personalized Herbal Diabetes Toolkit

Embarking on the journey of building your herbal diabetes toolkit requires a customized and well-informed strategy.

Developing Your Unique Herbal Plan

1. Recognizing Individual Needs: The Foundation of Personalization

Constructing a personalized herbal plan begins with a deep understanding of individual needs. Acknowledging the uniqueness of each person's diabetes journey involves tailoring herbal strategies to align with specific health objectives, preferences, and responses to herbs.

2. Defining Target Areas: Concentrating on Diabetes Management Goals

A personalized herbal plan involves a focused approach to diabetes management goals. Whether the emphasis is on blood sugar control, insulin sensitivity, or overall well-being, outlining specific objectives guides the selection of herbs that resonate with individual priorities.

3. Collaboration with Healthcare Professionals: Informed Decision-Making

In the creation of a personalized herbal plan, collaborating with healthcare professionals is pivotal. Transparent communication about herbal intentions ensures that chosen herbs complement existing treatment regimens, minimizing risks and maximizing therapeutic benefits.

4. Precision in Dosage and Administration

Personalizing an herbal plan extends to meticulous dosage considerations. Grasping the recommended dosages for chosen herbs and formulating a schedule that suits individual routines contributes to the precision and effectiveness of the herbal approach.

5. Holistic Integration into Lifestyle

Building a personalized herbal plan involves seamlessly integrating herbs into daily life. This holistic approach includes incorporating herbs into dietary habits, incorporating herbal teas, and exploring methods that align with an individual's lifestyle for sustained and practical application.

Reliable Sources for Obtaining Premium-Quality Herbs

1. Trustworthy Herbal Suppliers: Ensuring Quality and Purity

The core of a robust herbal toolkit lies in sourcing herbs from trustworthy suppliers. Identifying and selecting suppliers with a proven track record of quality, purity, and ethical standards is crucial. Researching supplier practices and customer reviews facilitates informed decisions about the reliability of herbal products.

2. Certifications and Standards: Ensuring Quality Assurance

Choosing herbs with recognized certifications and adherence to industry standards is a key consideration. Certifications such as organic, non-GMO, and Good Manufacturing Practices (GMP) provide assurance of quality and ethical sourcing practices, contributing to the overall integrity of the herbal toolkit.

3. Local Herbal Markets: Exploring Community Resources

Local herbal markets and community-based resources offer opportunities to connect directly with growers and suppliers. This direct interaction not only fosters community but also provides transparency in sourcing practices, enabling individuals to make informed choices about the quality of herbs in their toolkit.

4. Educational Platforms: Enhancing Knowledge and Awareness

Building an herbal toolkit is enriched by continuous learning. Engaging with educational platforms, such as workshops, seminars, and online courses, offers insights into herbal properties, applications, and responsible use. This knowledge empowers individuals to make informed decisions when selecting herbs for their personalized plan.

5. Herbalist Consultations: Professional Guidance

Consulting with herbalists provides a personalized and professional perspective on building an effective herbal toolkit. Herbalists can offer tailored advice based on individual health profiles, ensuring that chosen herbs align with specific needs and complement existing diabetes management strategies.

6. Online Herbal Communities: Shared Experiences and Recommendations

Online herbal communities provide platforms for individuals to share experiences and recommendations. Participating in these communities allows individuals to gain insights into effective herbs, dosage regimens, and potential challenges. This shared knowledge contributes to informed decision-making when selecting herbs for a personalized diabetes toolkit.

7. Herbal Gardens and Home Cultivation: Cultivating Quality

For those inclined toward a hands-on approach, cultivating herbs in home gardens provides a direct and quality-controlled source. Herbal gardens allow individuals to nurture herbs under specific conditions, ensuring freshness and potency in the herbs incorporated into their diabetes toolkit.

Concluding insights

In conclusion, crafting a personalized herbal plan and sourcing high-quality herbs are essential components of building a robust diabetes toolkit. Personalization involves understanding individual needs, setting specific goals, collaborating with healthcare professionals, and integrating herbs into daily life. Sourcing high-quality herbs entails selecting reputable suppliers, verifying certifications, exploring local markets, engaging with educational platforms, consulting herbalists, participating in online communities, and considering home cultivation. As individuals navigate this journey, the synergy of a personalized herbal plan and access to high-quality herbs creates a dynamic and empowering toolkit for managing diabetes effectively and holistically.

FAQs on Herbal Remedies for Diabetes

Embarking on the exploration of herbal remedies for diabetes triggers a multitude of questions. In this section, I address frequently asked questions (FAQs) surrounding the use of herbal remedies in diabetes management, providing clarity, evidence-based insights, and practical guidance.

Grasping Diabetes and the Role of Herbal Solutions

1. Defining Diabetes and Its Impact on the Body

Diabetes, characterized by elevated blood sugar levels, disrupts the body's insulin production or response. Herbal remedies play a role in managing blood sugar levels by targeting various pathways involved in glucose metabolism.

2. How Herbal Solutions Can Enhance Conventional Diabetes Treatments

Herbal remedies complement conventional treatments by offering additional support in blood sugar regulation, insulin sensitivity, and overall well-being. When used judiciously and in collaboration with healthcare professionals, herbs become valuable allies in comprehensive diabetes management.

Varieties, Causes, and Symptoms of Diabetes

1. Understanding the Diverse Types of Diabetes

Diabetes encompasses several types, including Type 1, Type 2, gestational diabetes, and prediabetes. Each type has distinct characteristics, and herbal remedies may be tailored to address specific needs associated with each type.

2. Addressing the Causes of Diabetes with Herbal Solutions

Diabetes has various causes, including genetic factors, lifestyle choices, and metabolic conditions. Herbal remedies may contribute to managing underlying causes by addressing inflammation, oxidative stress, and insulin resistance.

3. Recognizing Common Symptoms of Diabetes

Common symptoms, such as increased thirst, frequent urination, unexplained weight loss, fatigue, and blurred vision, may be alleviated by herbal remedies that promote better blood sugar control and overall metabolic health.

Efficacy and Safety of Herbal Remedies

1. Commonly Used Herbs for Diabetes and Their Mechanisms of Action

Herbs like aloe vera, bitter melon, fenugreek, cinnamon, gymnema sylvestre, and turmeric are common in diabetes management. They may work by enhancing insulin sensitivity, reducing blood sugar levels, and exerting anti-inflammatory effects.

2. Scientific Evidence Supporting Herbal Remedies for Diabetes

Scientific studies support the efficacy of certain herbs in diabetes management, highlighting their potential to improve glycemic control, modulate insulin activity, and offer antioxidant benefits. Individual responses may vary, necessitating consultation with healthcare professionals.

3. Safety Considerations and Possible Side Effects of Herbal Remedies

While many herbal remedies are generally safe, potential side effects and interactions exist. Consultation with healthcare professionals is crucial to ensure cautious and informed use, as some herbs may interact with medications or cause allergic reactions.

Integrating Herbal Remedies into Daily Life

1. Creating a Personalized Herbal Plan for Diabetes Management

Creating a personalized herbal plan involves understanding individual needs, collaborating with healthcare professionals, and integrating herbs into daily routines. The plan should consider specific diabetes management goals, dosage precision, and lifestyle integration.

2. Combining Herbal Remedies with Conventional Medications

Combining herbs with medications requires careful consideration and collaboration with healthcare providers. Open communication ensures a balanced and safe approach, as some herbs may interact with medications, affecting their efficacy or causing adverse effects.

3. Guidelines for Dosage and Administration of Herbal Remedies

Dosage guidelines vary for different herbs and depend on individual factors. It's essential to follow recommended dosages and administration methods. Healthcare professionals can offer personalized guidance based on health status and treatment goals.

Addressing Challenges and Taking Precautions

1. Precautions for Individuals with Diabetes Using Herbal Remedies

Individuals with diabetes should consult healthcare professionals before incorporating herbal remedies. Monitoring blood sugar levels, being aware of potential interactions, and promptly reporting any adverse effects are essential precautions.

2. Herbal Remedies for Pregnant Individuals with Diabetes

Pregnant individuals with diabetes should exercise heightened caution and consult healthcare professionals before using herbal remedies. Individualized guidance is crucial as some herbs may pose risks during pregnancy.

3. Herbal Remedies for Children with Diabetes
The use of herbal remedies in children with diabetes requires careful consideration. Dosages should be adjusted based on age and weight, and healthcare professionals should be consulted to ensure safety and efficacy.

Herbal Remedies: Beyond Blood Sugar Control

1. Overall Well-being with Herbal Remedies

Certain herbs have properties that contribute to overall well-being. Anti-inflammatory and antioxidant effects may enhance cardiovascular health and reduce diabetes-related complications.

2. Timeline for Results with Herbal Remedies

Individual responses vary, and the time to see results with herbal remedies depends on factors such as the herb used, dosage, and overall health. Consistency in usage, coupled with lifestyle modifications, contributes to optimal results.

3. Duration of Herbal Use

The duration of herbal use depends on individual needs and responses. Periodic assessments with healthcare professionals guide adjustments to the herbal plan based on changing health conditions and treatment goals.

Future Avenues and Research

1. Current Research on Herbal Remedies for Diabetes

Ongoing research explores the potential of herbal compounds in diabetes management.

Scientific investigations aim to uncover new insights into mechanisms of action, paving the way for innovative and evidence-based herbal interventions.

2. Integration of Herbal Approaches in Diabetes Care at Integrative Clinics

Integrative clinics are increasingly incorporating herbal approaches into diabetes care. Interdisciplinary teams of healthcare professionals collaborate to provide comprehensive strategies that combine conventional and herbal treatments.

Concluding insights

In conclusion, addressing FAQs on herbal remedies for diabetes empowers individuals with knowledge, dispels misconceptions, and fosters informed choices. Collaboration with healthcare professionals, adherence to safety precautions, and a commitment to personalized and evidence-based approaches contribute to holistic well-being. The synergy between scientific understanding and traditional wisdom creates a dynamic framework for managing diabetes effectively and proactively with herbal remedies.

Conclusion

As I conclude this expedition, let's encapsulate key insights:

Grasping Diabetes and Herbal Remedies

✔ Diabetes Clarified: Diabetes, marked by elevated blood sugar levels, disrupts the body's insulin production or response.

✔ Herbal Synergy: Herbal remedies complement conventional treatments by supporting blood sugar regulation and overall well-being.

Types, Causes, and Symptoms of Diabetes

✔ Diverse Diabetes Types: From Type 1 to

gestational diabetes, each type requires

tailored approaches.

✔ Herbal Contributions to Causes: Herbal

remedies may contribute to managing

underlying causes like inflammation

and insulin resistance.

✔ Recognizing Symptoms: Identifying

common symptoms allows for targeted

herbal interventions.

Efficacy and Safety of Herbal Remedies

✔ Herbs in Focus: Aloe vera, bitter melon,

   fenugreek, cinnamon, gymnema

   sylvestre, and turmeric are herbs with

   potential benefits for diabetes.

✔ Scientific Backing: Studies support the

   efficacy of certain herbs in improving

   glycemic control and insulin activity.

✔ Safety Emphasis: While generally safe,

   herbal remedies require caution and

   consultation with healthcare

   professionals.

Integrating Herbal Remedies into Daily Life

✔ Personalized Plans: Creating a personalized herbal plan involves understanding needs, collaborating with healthcare professionals, and integrating herbs into routines.

✔ Harmony with Medications: Combining herbs with medications requires careful consideration and open communication.

✔ Precision in Dosage: Adherence to precise dosages and administration methods enhances herbal remedy effectiveness.

Addressing Challenges and Taking Precautions

✔ Precautions for Individuals: Caution, monitoring, and prompt reporting are essential for individuals incorporating herbal remedies.

✔ Special Populations Consideration: Pregnant individuals and children with diabetes require specialized guidance and precautions.

✔ Herbal Remedies: Beyond Blood Sugar Control

✔ Overall Well-being: Some herbs contribute to overall well-being with anti-inflammatory and antioxidant effects.

✔ Results and Duration: Consistent use and lifestyle modifications contribute to optimal results, and the duration of herbal use depends on individual needs.

Future Avenues and Research

✔ Ongoing Research: Continuous research

explores the potential of herbal

compounds in diabetes management.

✔ Clinics' Integrative Approaches:

Integrative clinics increasingly

incorporate herbal approaches into

diabetes care.

Embracing Holistic Diabetes Management

As we reflect on this wealth of information,

the call to embrace a holistic approach to

diabetes management becomes paramount.

The harmonious integration of herbal remedies with conventional treatments offers a nuanced and personalized strategy for individuals navigating the complexities of diabetes.

The significances include:

1. Empowerment in Wellness Planning: The essence of a holistic approach lies in empowering individuals to create personalized wellness plans. Understanding individual needs, setting specific goals, and collaborating with healthcare professionals facilitate a tailored diabetes management strategy.

2. Collaborative Healthcare Partnership: The journey toward holistic diabetes management involves a strong partnership with healthcare professionals. Open communication, regular check-ins, and transparent sharing of herbal plans ensure interventions align with overall health goals and existing medical conditions.

3. Safety as the Cornerstone: Safety is paramount in the holistic management of diabetes. Whether incorporating herbal remedies, medications, or lifestyle modifications, prioritizing safety considerations through professional guidance

and vigilant self-monitoring becomes a shared responsibility.

4. Knowledge Empowerment: Knowledge serves as a powerful tool in the pursuit of holistic well-being. Educating individuals about the properties, benefits, and potential risks associated with herbal remedies empowers them to make informed decisions and actively participate in their health journey.

5. Consistency and Adaptability: Consistency in incorporating herbal remedies into daily life, coupled with adaptability to changing health conditions, forms the bedrock of

holistic diabetes management. Regular assessments, adjustments, and a dynamic approach contribute to sustained well-being.

6. Nurturing Overall Health: Holistic diabetes management transcends the singular focus on blood sugar control. It encompasses nurturing overall health, addressing inflammation, supporting cardiovascular health, and mitigating diabetes-related complications.

7. Looking to the Future: The integration of herbal remedies into diabetes care is an evolving field. Ongoing research promises exciting possibilities, paving the way for new insights, innovations, and evidence-based

interventions that could reshape the landscape of diabetes management.

Embracing a holistic approach to diabetes management signifies a commitment to comprehensive well-being. By combining the wisdom of herbal remedies with the expertise of healthcare professionals, individuals embark on a journey that transcends symptom control, aiming for a life rich in vitality and balanced health. As we move forward, let the synergy of traditional wisdom and scientific understanding guide us toward a future where holistic diabetes management becomes not just a strategy but a way of life.